From a wheelchair to working

Lyme no longer controls my life

"She begins to heal"

1

For Donna

You taught me to live even when I felt like I was dying. You showed me what true friendship was. I hope you're singing and decorating in heaven.

Notice

The protocols, the medicine I describe in this book, should in no way be taken for medical advice. I am not a doctor; I am just giving suggestions of things to investigate.

I Hope you never….

I hope you never wake up one day and can't walk.

I hope you never feel so scared because you don't know what is happening to you.

I hope you never have to see over thirty-five doctors because your so sick, but they don't believe you. because you look fine.

I hope you never have to sit in an office crying begging a doctor to help you only to be told it's all in your head.

I hope you never get embarrassed because you can no longer speak right because your brain is full of fog.

I hope you never have to prove to your partner that you are truly sick, and hope they believe you this time.

I hope you never feel so alone, looking out at the world wondering how you go to this place in your life.

I hope you never have to fake it, so your family doesn't get sick of you not feeling well.

I hope you never have to give up your hopes and dreams.

I hope you never have to lose people you love because they just don't understand how bad it gets.

I hope you never feel guilty because you got sick.

I hope you never get Lyme Disease.

Table of contents

Chapter 1 -The Aftermath

Chapter 2- Toxins and environmental triggers MCAS or Mass Cell

Chapter 3-Lyme bill

Chapter 4-Infectious Disease Doctor

Chapter 5- Obtaining my degree and moving forward with my health

Chapter 6-Seizures, Scented Chemicals, and Mold Illness and Ebv

Chapter 7-Diet and exercise

Chapter 8-Lyme protocols

Chapter 9-Burning Mouth Syndrome

Chapter 10- Disulfiram

Chapter 11- Here and Now

Chapter 12- The Coronavirus

Chapter 13-Living with Lyme

Please note if you are newly bit seek medical treatment right away. At least three to four weeks of antibiotics, me personally would get at least six weeks for a new bite. The protocols in this book is things you can do when treatment wasn't given right away, (within a few weeks or so of the bite). Or if you weren't properly treated.

Chapter 1

The aftermath from our first book.

If you read my first book titled "From a wheelchair to walking, one person's Lyme story in Illinois" you know that Lyme put me through hell. Throughout this whole process, I sometimes felt like I was on a roller-coaster that I never asked to be on, but I couldn't get off no matter how hard I tried. In the beginning, I felt like I was being punished, I mean, why else would I be given this horrible, complicated disease? If I was to be given a disease, I thought at least give me one that people know about. In 2012 no one knew about Lyme; I was constantly having to prove to everyone that I was sick. It was a nightmare.

Then I started to think maybe I was given this disease because I wouldn't just sit back and take it. I would do my best to do something about it. That is why I had my daughter help me with the first book, to let others know they are not alone. In 2012 I felt completely alone. Once the book was finished and out there, I had some good responses and some not so great ones. One person told me that I was going to just die anyway, and at first, that response hurt me. I spent every single day trying to find the strength in me to keep fighting. To tell someone that is fighting to live that they are just going to die is rough to hear. I was also told that there is no point in treating Lyme since we don't have a cure for it yet.

For me, not treating is not an option, even if that means I have to self-treat. If I don't treat my symptoms, they get so bad that I can't walk. My body turns to concrete. I find that I get dizzy, and my brain gets a burning sensation so intense that I feel like my head is going to explode. This is not a headache or a migraine, it's more like brain zaps, or the nerves in my brain being set on fire. The seizures get so bad that I can't do anything but lay in bed. In my opinion, and I am not a doctor or a medical professional, we have to treat this disease, even if we do it our way. I had a few people say the first book did not give a set protocol, and I agree because there is not one. I list things that I felt helped me, and I feel may help others, but I can't tell people what to buy or what to take. With Lyme, we are all different. We have different strands, different co-infections, the only thing I can do is make suggestions for a person to investigate. I hope that it may help you as it has me.

I want to thank every single person that brought our first book. I have made it my goal to turn what happened to me into something positive. This last year I have been looking at my life and some of the things that I have gone through. In the last few weeks, I have been thinking that one reason that I have not completely healed from Lyme is that I have suffered so much trauma in my life. I had a rough childhood, and without boring everyone with the details there was a lot of violence and abuse. When I became a parent. I honestly did not know what I was doing. I know I wasn't the best parent to my children. I yelled a lot, and I didn't have much patience. Looking back now, in a way we take parts of our childhood with us as we become parents. This last year I am trying to be a better parent, and a better person. I know that can be difficult when we are fighting a disease like Lyme, but we must try.

I feel like I need to say that I have Lyme Disease, but I am not Lyme Disease. When I first became sick the disease took over every thought that I had. I gave so much power to the disease because I didn't know any other way. I didn't understand what was happening to me, and so many people in my life did not understand it either. We still do not completely understand this disease, I feel like we are still learning, and the world is still learning too though. There are still times when I have a rough day, but now I consider that a bad symptom day or a flare-up day. I tell myself this so that my mind knows this is only temporary.

I had quite a few people ask me how I get through this because it's so painful, so overwhelming. I allow my body to rest when I am tired now. I'll still turn to something I love like music when things get rough. I have found that I can read again where in the past I couldn't because my eyes would get so blurry. So, I go to the library which has always been one of my favorite places and I take out a few books. Or I watch a funny movie. Anything to take my mind off the disease for a while. To me you must find what makes you happy, and it could be something as simple as watching the sunrise or smelling the rain. Whatever it is that gives peace to your soul.

When I was stuck in bed and couldn't walk, I made a promise to myself that if I ever found a way out I would share it. I would talk about it so much people would get sick of hearing it. Are you sick of hearing about it yet? I hope not. This is a journey, and not just my journey. It's a journey for millions of people like me going through the same disease. I still think that we all can get into remission. We just have to find what works for us, and honestly for me, I am never going to stop trying. I am getting there but it's slow, and for someone like me patience isn't my thing so that is hard. I want the magic pill, the magic protocol that just doesn't exist yet. There are things to make us feel better or to calm our symptoms, but the truth is we are probably always going to have Lyme. So we need to find a way to calm our symptoms down enough that we can live with it. Even though I have been through all of this I still find life to be a beautiful thing. I still get excited when the seasons change and when the flowers bloom.

Once the book was published I was asked to give two speeches: one was at a Lyme walk here in Illinois. I am not a great public speaker, but I did it to offer people hope. A few years ago I was so sick I couldn't even put my socks on, and now I am walking on my own. At one time I had to crawl to the washroom so many times that I lost count. I can tell you if you're reading this, there is something so humbling about not being able to walk, and then one day you can again. It's almost like I was given a second chance at life. So, if I can help one person not go through six years of this like I had to, then it's been worth it to me.

I see things much more differently than I did before. I can't allow negative things or negative people to get into my head, to get into my heart. If I am going to heal, truly heal, I need to let things go. I need to find a way to release the trauma that I have experienced in my life and this is something I am working on every day. It's very difficult to go from working and providing to being unemployed. It takes away a person's self-esteem when something like this happens, and it brought back so many fears and doubts I had my whole life. It's something personally I must work on. At the end of the day, I am doing the best I can.

It would be easy to stay angry, but I can't allow anger to control my life anymore. Having a disease like Lyme has taught me compassion, that in the past I never really had. I used to have to prove to people that I was sick, and I don't any longer. I don't need anyone to believe me anymore. I found that I can't change what people think of me. After a while you will probably get to this point too. If they don't understand or they don't have compassion, then screw them. Seriously trying to prove to people that do not want to hear you takes too much time, and too much energy. That energy can be spent on healing.

Chapter 2

Toxins and environmental triggers

MCAS or Mast Cell

At some point, I started to realize that certain toxins in my environment were making so many of us sick. I feel that Lyme, parasites, and mold started this and made most of our bodies hypersensitive. Some people can't even be around Wi-Fi as they react. For me, I react to things like dryer sheets, perfume, laundry soap, and glade plugins. If I get around any of these things my body starts to burn; my face will start to turn red and I will most likely go into a seizure. Also, candles will force my body into tremors where in the past I could be around all of these things no problem. I found one of the worst triggers to be around is the spray that goes on lawns for pests. These are used mostly everywhere; in our local stores we shop in, on grass when we walk down the street, even some doctor's offices have scented objects. So how do we heal when the environment that we live in is making us sick?

I have been asking myself this question for over six years. Since we can't control our environment we need to try and control how our bodies react to them. I first learned of Mast Cell disorder when my daughter became sick last year. She was working at a local department store that sold perfume and she started to get hives. At first, it was just a few hives. Then the hives spread all over her body, and bruises started to appear. We took her to all the doctors we could, and no one could tell us what was wrong with her. They kept saying she has allergies, but that didn't explain the hives to me. So I started to research, and I learned about mass cell disorder. I found out that we had to have her on two different antihistamines to control her body from having a histamine reaction. We use Zyrtec/Zantac combo and had to go up on the doses until her hives were under control. This took us almost a year, but then we found an allergist in Morton Grove that listened to us and diagnosed her with Mast Cell Disorder.

Here is my daughter during one of her outbreaks.

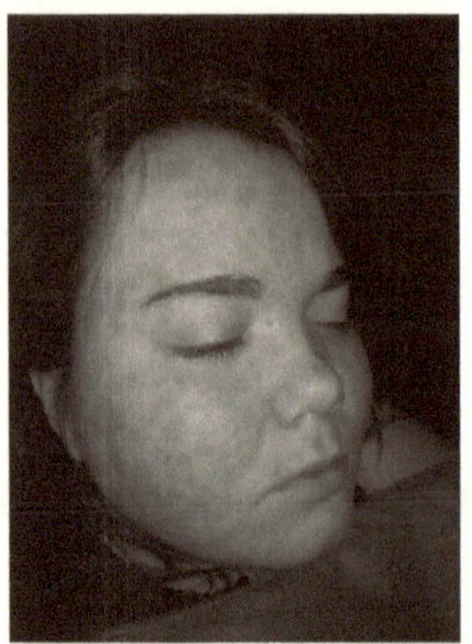

     Mast cell activation **syndrome** (MCAS) is one type of **mast cell** activation **disorder** (MCAD) and is an immunological condition in which **mast cells** inappropriately and excessively release chemical mediators, resulting in a range of chronic **symptoms**, sometimes including anaphylaxis or near-anaphylaxis attacks.

     If you don't know how dangerous this is, one day she woke up and she couldn't breathe. Her body was covered head to toe with these hives. Her throat was closing, I had to call an ambulance to get her to the hospital. She became allergic to everything. Every day it was a new allergy, or a different food. For instance, today, she could be allergic to pineapple, tomorrow it would be something else like lettuce. She had to take a leave from her college classes and quit her job. It took us over a year to get her where she can eat most foods or go into a public place without getting these reactions.

     Now for me, I don't get the hives, I get neurological symptoms when I am exposed. I started mast-ease a few months ago. It helps with some of the symptoms but does not stop all the symptoms. I still have to wear a mask if I go to the laundromat because all those chemicals make me sick. I am still trying to find a way to completely control all the symptoms, and that is a never-ending process. It's not one thing that is making us sick, it's not just the Lyme. I think the Lyme turned our bodies on to be overly sensitive to everything.

I watched the mold summit and they mentioned a product found on amazon. It's called Amazing Nutrition- Quercetin 800 Mg with Bromelain 165 Mg, I started taking this daily. I am going to work up to the recommended three times a day. I had to start slow and my body reacts poorly to most things. I am seeing some positive changes with this medicine. I spilled some blcach the other day, and I normally would have seized from that in the past. I would have started to burn, like smelling the bleach would get so deep inside me that it would feel as if it was poured inside my brain. I did not react; I was able to clean it up without an issue.

Then yesterday, I was walking up the backstairs and someone in my building was using scented dryer sheets. Now this has always been a huge trigger for me. I smelt it and just kept going. I was waiting for my body to start to seize and it did not. This tells me that using medicine to lower my mast cells is helping me. I hope to one day not react at all, no matter what the chemical is. I am not there yet, but I am working towards it now. I do not believe it's just the one medicine alone. I think doing the Biocidin with it is helping me to detox the mold and to bust open the biofilm.

Chapter 3

Lyme bills for Illinois

I was extremely upset when part of the Lyme bill was vetoed by the governor, the part that allowed long term treatment to Lyme patients. I am happy to say that the bill has been since overturned and will be a law as of January 2019. This is amazing news for everyone suffering from Lyme and could not have happened without the legislators here helping by co-sponsoring this bill.

When I first became sick in 2012 and realized how hard it was to get treatment here I reached out to every senator I could, even the president. At that time, not too many people were sick with Lyme, so they did not take me seriously. Now fast forward to 2019, and we have thousands of people, thousands of families sick. This upsets me because this could have been avoided if they would have listened to me back when I tried to tell them. Sometimes I think did I try hard enough? I mean, I was so sick I could barely sit up, but I could still write and call people asking for help with this disease.

Now we are in 2020 and there is not only one Lyme bill in place but there are two. The first bill Hb4115 was put in place to protect our doctors from treating us. This was brought about because of a very young warrior here in Illinois and her mom that is amazing. We now have a law that states Lyme patients must be covered for treatment with insurance. When I first became sick, I had the best insurance money could buy. I remember calling to try and get IV antibiotics and I was told the insurance wouldn't cover it. I would have to pay 10,000 out of pocket for it.

This was at the time that I had gone from full time to part-time. I was losing my house that had black mold and we needed to find a place to live as soon as possible. I often think back to that day if insurance would have helped me, or if anyone would have helped me here, I know I would not have become as sick. I am not saying people didn't help me, my family, my kids, my husband did. I mean actual medical professionals. If they would have stepped in to help me, instead of saying I was crazy maybe the last 6 or 7 years would have been different? I try to not dwell on 'what ifs.' It's hard because I had a good accounting career that I had worked my whole life for. I lost everything to Lyme for a long time.

When I think about the first four or five years I am not even sure how we made it. How did I even survive? I want you to imagine having 20 plus seizures a day and going to the doctor after doctor begging for help. Then I want you to imagine a doctor telling you were crazy, that there wasn't Lyme in Illinois. How would you feel? Or take your caregiver in another room, the only person that is paying for you to survive, to have them tell you that you could stop all of this if you really wanted to. I was treated horrible. Patients with Lyme are treated horribly. No one should be treated this way. If anything at all comes from my story it's I hope that people see Lyme differently. I hope they understand how bad it is, how bad it can be. We continue to lose Lyme patients all over the country because they can't get proper treatment, and because of how people in the medical community have treated us. We have families giving up on their family members over Lyme, leaving them to their own suffering and fight for themselves. This should never happen, yet it does every single day.

Chapter 4

Infectious Disease Doctor

On December 13th, 2018 I started to see an infectious disease doctor in Elgin. On the way to my first appointment, I was so nervous I tried to talk myself out of going. If you have Lyme or know someone with Lyme, they will understand this. We with Lyme are sometimes treated so badly that a new doctor will give us PTSD. I was so nervous I almost threw up in the car. The last infectious disease doctor wrote up a paper saying I needed to be put into a mental institution because I had my positive Lyme test on me at the hospital. I was told before going that this doctor would be different, he had Lyme, so he understood.

When the doctor walked into the room, I took a deep breath and told my story. He asked questions and listened to me. After hearing my story, he said I think you have Bart, a coinfection plus Lyme. He said we are going to run some tests, and we are going to start treating. I was in shock, he did not think I was crazy and he knew that I was sick. He warned me that once we started treating the infections, I would get worse before I got better. He started me on a month of Azithromycin, then a month of doxy. When I was put on the doxy my left knee swelled up twice it's size. The doctor said I don't have to run any more tests, that is a clear indicator you still have Lyme in your body.

Around the 2nd month when I was almost finished with the doxy, I went into a bad herx. I was trying to cook breakfast and suddenly my brain started to burn badly. (I attribute this to die off in the brain). My body can't detox on its own, since I have two of the MTHFR genes. I was holding my head, and just pacing back and forth in my kitchen. It sounds crazy now saying this, but my brain was saying go outside. Now at the time it was the middle of winter in Illinois, and we were having a really cold winter, and I was getting ready to go outside. I began to look for my shoes, kind of disoriented. My husband noticed what I was doing and told me to stay inside. The only thing outside by me is the train behind my house. I want to say this: before Lyme I was never suicidal, and I never had these kinds of thoughts. Since getting Lyme and co-infections, sometimes my thoughts are so bad, so scary, it frightens me. I will get random thoughts like you're never going to get better; your family is going to get sick of you being sick and leave you. You're a burden, you can't even work, you're a loser. These were the thoughts that would pop in my head, and even worse ones like 'no one would care if you died', and 'you would be doing everyone in your life a favor' would pop up.

16

It's like I am in a constant battle with good and evil, with the evil being the Lyme. I sometimes feel like my body, my whole life, is at war. I am fighting a war inside myself. It's hard to explain, but I think that is why there is such a high percentage of suicide amongst Lyme patients. I feel tick-borne diseases like Lyme trigger mental illness. I never had depression in my life until I got sick with Lyme. Afterwards, I was extremely anxious all the time. I think the isolation, the inability to work, and the stigma causes depression. I was having a conversation with another Lyme patient and we both agreed that Lyme it's like being trapped in your own body. I have said this before; we want to do things like work and socialize, but our bodies won't cooperate. I can be planning to go somewhere, maybe the store for groceries, and my body will randomly start having tremors, and then I'm stuck in bed. This is happening less and less now that I am aggressively treating the disease, but it will forever stink that sometimes I will still have to cancel things due to my health issues.

After two months of oral antibiotics, the ID doctor decided I needed to do a PICC line. The insurance would cover 28 days of iv rocephin. My husband kept asking me if I was sure I wanted to do this. I mean, I never treated Lyme with Iv antibiotics so we were not sure how my body would react. My doctor had me on orals for two months to get my body ready for it. I was told the PICC line does not hurt, but I found this to be false for me. It turns out I have a ton of nerve clusters in my arm and the nurses had no choice but to go through them to get to the heart… Yes, as you imagine, it was painful.

The way my insurance is set up, I have Medicare. They would give me the antibiotics, but I would have to go to the hospital in Elk Grove every single day for 28 days to get my treatment. This made me nervous. In the past, hospitals have not been nice to me, so many of them did not understand Lyme and I was treated like either a crazy person. The first time I walked into the ambulatory care unit, the vibe inside was really good. People seemed to be busy, but happy, and I kind of picked up on that.

I was treated very well there the whole 28 days, not one issue. When I had two small seizures they rushed me to the ER there. I was nervous again; PTSD I think from bad medical treatment in the past. The ER treated me very well too, the nurse said her best friend has Lyme, so she understands. That was super sweet to have someone that understands how bad it can get.

Chapter 5

Obtaining a degree and moving forward

I am not sure if I mentioned this is the first book, but I suffered brain damage from a seizure around 2015/2016. The neurologist at the time told me I wouldn't be able to do the job that I once had in accounting because the part of my brain that calculates math was affected. I have been trying to finish college, my associate degree, for almost 10 years. I had to drop out three times due to my Lyme Disease. I am very excited to say on August 5th of 2019, I received my diploma.

After finally getting my diploma I have decided to go back to school and get my bachelor's degree in human services with a focus on psychology. When I first became sick no one understood what I was going through. I didn't know of any therapist that understood Lyme and understood the anxiety that goes with it. So, in September 2019, I will start an online course. I am excited and I want to help people that have disabilities and that become disabled.

In September 2019, I started going to NLU (National Louis University) to get my human service degree. The whole degree will be online for me which is very important while I am going through Lyme and mold treatment. I can't do more than one class at a time per my doctor's orders. I never thought I would be able to do this, after my health failed so bad in 2012, by the time we were in 2014/2015 I didn't think I was going to survive. Those years were bad years for me, traumatic and painful. In my head, I always told myself I could get better if I just figured out how to.

I still watch all the summits for Lyme, mold, or whatever I can get my hands on and take notes. I realized a long time ago that we had to be our advocate, there was no one to come and save us so we had to save ourselves. For a long time I was very angry and upset about what happened to me. I had to realize I could hold on to that anger and be miserable, or I could take that anger and turn it into something positive like helping others with this disease. So that is what I try to do, be a positive force in the Lyme community.

Even though I now have more good days than bad I still have days when I have a seizure and my body just locks up. My recovery time is quite a bit better now, but it has become my mission to make sure I get these seizures to stop. I realized recently since I have had Lyme I have been diagnosed with having pleurisy six times. For people that do not know Pleurisy is an inflammation of the lung lining. The severity of the condition can range from mild to life-threatening. It's very painful.

On September 1st, 2019, I started to have bad chest pain, it felt like someone was stabbing me. It would come and go, and I keep hoping it would go away so I didn't have to go to the hospital. By September 2nd the pain was so bad I couldn't take it anymore. We tend to go to the big hospital in Downers Grove as they have always treated me very well. I am sure you understand why it's so important to somewhere that you feel safe.

After an EKG , X-ray, and some blood tests, the ER doctor told me he thought it was Pleurisy again. He gave me IV medicine, a non-steroid kind because he felt with steroids it could cause the Lyme in my body to go crazy. The hospital there seems to be learning more and more about Lyme. They have never once mistreated me. He suggested I see a cardiologist, so I made an appointment, they were able to get me in the very next day. The cardiologist I saw was amazing, I mean even her nurse said it takes a very long time to recover from Lyme. They seem to understand how bad this disease can be.

The doctor suggests I have an echo to check the pleurisy and to also see if Lyme has damaged anything in my heart. Originally, I was having that, and a heart monitor was to be put in on October 1st. Today, which is September 5th, I woke up feeling okay, but by 8 am I was in horrible pain again. I called the office back, and the lady answering the phone said I can tell you're in pain by your voice lets see what we can do for you. They moved all my appointments up, so tomorrow I will have the echo and the heart monitor. Everything was normal so I followed up with my Lyme doctor. We talked about pleurisy and the fact that I have mycoplasma. He believes this could be causing some of my issues with my chest, so we are treating with Clindamycin.

I was able to get through that and start to feel better. With Lyme it comes and goes so with many different symptoms. It's hard to tell sometimes if this is heart-related, Lyme related, or co-infections. I try not to go to the hospital unless it gets really bad where I feel like I have no other choice then I will go.

Chapter 6

Seizures and Scented chemicals and Mold and Ebv

We have finally figured out what is causing my seizures: it's anything chemically scented. If I use a shampoo that has a scent in it, I will seize. If I go into a store or doctor's office and they have a plugin that sprays scented stuff, I will seize within a few minutes. It has become so bad that when I went into a dollar store the other day, I was literally in there for like five minutes, I seized. As I was trying to walk out, I started to slur my words, stubble, and looked like a drunk person. By the time I made it to our truck, I started to go into a spasm, when I sat down my husband said he knew they were coming. I had a couple of bad seizures and then my legs locked up.

When I got home, I said I had enough, I need to get this taken care of. I started looking for doctors that knew about mold, and seizures. I thought I found a great one. I researched him first and watched some of his videos. He seemed really smart, a little dry humored, but smart. He's in California, and he treats people all over the United States. I had a few hundred dollars saved up, so I gave him a call. The first call he was nice and seemed like he was going to help me. The 2nd call, he said what's your problem, you sound young. I said I am 43 years old, I have Lyme, and before I was able to finish he said 'well, everyone thinks they have Lyme.' I took a deep breath because I was not having it, I said well I have a positive western blot and was just treated by an infectious disease doctor. Then his attitude changed some but at this point, I was already done with him. He wanted 600 bucks a month to try and help me. There is no way I could afford that and told him that. Some of these so-called doctors are just taking advantage of sick people.

I am not sure how much of this I mentioned in the first Lyme book, but I also suffer from mold illness, or what is also called sick building syndrome. I bought a house in 2008 that contained five different types of mold, but the worst was that it contained what is known as the black mold. Its full name is Stachybotrys chartarum, when we brought the house it passed the FHA inspection because the mold was in the walls and under the floors. We were not aware of this until I started getting sick. Also, I worked in a place that flooded at least 3 or 4 times while I was there. The workers helped clean up and were later working in a very moldy environment. At this time, I did not know anything about mold or what it could due to a person, especially a person like me that can't detox it. In the first book, I mentioned I can't detox on my own because of two MTHFR genes that I carry. So, when I get exposed to something as bad as mold, I can't get it out of the body and it just sits there causing me to get sicker and sicker.

I have been looking for a mold doctor for the last few years. The ones I have found here are so expensive I could not afford them. I also have been watching the Mold summits online and taking notes. I have always felt that mold was a huge issue for me, I just didn't know how to fix it. We are now in September of 2019, and my husband suggested I look for an environmental doctor that specializes in environmental illness. So, I went to a site for people suffering from mcas and came across a student here in Illinois that was studying environmental issues. I figured I would give her a call and see if she knew someone that could help me. I told her that I believe I am suffering from mold illness and asked her if she knew of any doctor that could help me. She told me about a medical facility here in my town that has a doctor that knows about mold and Lyme.

I called and made an appointment. I was extremely nervous going into the appointment. I had my folder with me, my positive Lyme test, some blood work and I dressed up. Let's face it, as a woman going into a doctor's office at times we are treated differently in some cases than how men are treated. I feel like from the moment the doctor walks into the room we are being judged. I know that sounds a little crazy, but it has happened to me over and over. Now I am a different person, and I told my husband if I walk in and the doctor treats me like I am either crazy or exaggerating we are leaving.

We walked into the waiting room, filled out some paperwork, and were told to be seated so that someone would be there shortly. We just waited a few minutes as we were early, then doctor interns showed up to take us to a room. They were younger doctors in training, and I did not feel uncomfortable talking to them. We then spent about 3 hours going over my medical history, and my family history. They would leave the room at times to go and consult the head doctor there, the doctor I wanted to see. A few times she came into the room too to ask questions, or to see how we were doing. I explained that I am so sensitive to scented things that just going into a dollar store the week before caused me to have slurred speech, inability to walk right, and then two seizures. This is where the doctor in training surprised me, she said are you allergic to electric magnetic fields too, like wi-fi. I explained that I was not, she said that was good then.

The interns went to talk to Dr. G, and they all came back with a health plan. I looked at the paper and said, oh we are going after mold. I know I had seen the protocols before, but I have always felt I needed a doctor to guide me. During about 2014 I tried to treat mold with CSM by myself, and got so sick I was bedridden for 9 months. I can't do that again, I can't be bedridden, and I need a doctor to guide me. I know I have self-treated a lot over the years only because I had no other choice. I do not feel I would be alive today if I didn't. I was in bad shape. I mean at one time I was having whole days where I couldn't speak correctly, where I couldn't swallow, and I couldn't feed myself. I had what the doctor's thought was possibly ALS. It was not ALS, it was Lyme, co-infections and mold toxins destroying my body. I also think if someone is diagnosed with ALS, MS, Fibro, or a seizure disorder they should investigate tick-borne disease and mold illness.

Since I have gone the prescription route for mold before and it did not help me I have been looking for alternative treatment options. I watch mold summits as much as I can, and take notes. Even when I went to see the new set of doctors in my gut I knew that I would have to use a binder, and still use a product to open my pathways. This is my mold protocol, now I am in no way a doctor, I am only sharing this because I am on day two now, and I feel it's working for me. It may help someone else to try it.

Herbal treatment for Mold toxins in my body. This was given to me by an Np medical training office here in my town.

Biocidin to break up biofilm, one drops 3 time a day for one week, then add one drop per day.

Theracurmin Hp - 2 capsules a day for inflammation

Vital Nutrients liver support - 2 capsules a day for better liver detox

Fiber flows - 2 capsules a day for one week then goes up to 3 daily. To clear the liver and help consistently use the bathroom.

Fir Sauna - 2 times a week for 20 minutes then shower in cold water for 30 seconds. My daughter brought me a sauna from eBay. It works well. I put it on 140 temps, and sweat like crazy.

EBV

When I first became sick in 2012, my EBV or Epstein Barr numbers were over 600. Since then, we are now into 2019, my test in March of this year showed that my numbers were still 600. I started taking the biocidin and the mass cell medicine called quercetin bromelain, and from March to November my numbers dropped to 545. I will share a picture of each so you can see what I am talking about.

For me, fatigue has always been a huge issue since I got Lyme.

If I folded laundry, I would have to take breaks in between. I am not talking about just being tired, you know how your body feels like when you have the flu? That is how my body felt every single day, completely drained. As my numbers are starting to lower I am finding myself getting a little more energy. I also added doing the sauna twice a week, it's just a cheap one my daughter found on eBay, but it goes up to 140 degrees and it works.

My numbers are starting to go down. When our bodies are so full of viruses, parasites, mold, and Lyme it's hard to recover at all from anything. I am working hard every day to get this crap out of my body, but it's difficult.

Chapter 7

Diet and Exercise

When I first became sick each doctor told me I had to go on a different diet. I have tried most, if not all, diets. I went gluten-free for about 9 months because the doctor at the time thought it would cure my seizures, it did not. Then one doctor said I had to eat only raw foods, so I did it. I lasted a little over a week before getting even sicker. I found that a person with mold should not be on this diet. Then I did paleo, and finally ketogenic. Each time the doctors told me to do this or that, and I tried to follow it 100 percent. Right now, because of the mold, I am on a low sugar, low dairy diet. This one is not as bad as some of the others as I can still eat meat and fresh vegetables. I try to eat only non-GMO.

I remember way back in 2013/2014 when I was in a wheelchair and on a cane most of the time. I remember a doctor telling me to get on the floor and do yoga even though I could barely move. There were days I was crawling to do certain things. I remember being very upset and angry because I couldn't do what she asked. It felt like her telling me to do it meant she did not believe I was that sick.

Now we are into September 2019, and I can exercise some. I can walk around for about 15 to 20 minutes without collapsing now. When I first tried to use my treadmill I could only make it a minute or two. I had to use my arms to steady myself, and after two minutes I was done for the day. My primary had wanted me to do water therapy but because of my seizures I would always need a lifeguard. I couldn't get anyone to do that for me, so I decided to do my therapy at home.

This is important, when we are well enough, I think we should try and move some every day. Even if that means taking a five- or 15-minute walk. If you're new to Lyme this is not going to happen right away.

It has taken me over 7 years to finally be able to do this, but I'm doing it. When I was in the wheelchair I would do arm and leg weights. I did so so my body would not lose muscle. Keeping my body moving was so when I was able to I could walk right again.

Some days I would get up and my legs would move. Other days I would try to stand, and my legs would fold like noodles. This would happen over and over throughout the days and nights. I used to fall so much that if I had a day that I didn't fall I considered that a better day. So, the fact that I can exercise now is amazing, but this has not been a quick fix. It's been a slow and steady process, if I went too fast, I would get worse, so I now listen to my body.

We are now in March of 2020 and I can walk for 20 to 30 minutes at least 3 times a week. For someone that could only stand on a treadmill for a few minutes this is amazing. I am slowly trying to build my body up. If I am too tired I rest, but when I feel decent, I push my body to make it work. I think it's very important to get the body moving because if we don't use our muscles they start weakening. I learned that when I was bedridden. I would try and stretch my body and do a little exercise, but when you're stuck in bed that makes it very difficult.

Chapter 8

Lyme protocols

And a treatment plan

I am going to list the Lyme protocols that I am aware of here. I am only listing cheaper protocols that people can do if they can't afford to get an LLMD. Please know that as I said, in the beginning, I am in no way a doctor, and what I am referring to here can be found online. Each person should investigate them and talk to a physician if possible before treating. If you can't afford a doctor, I will share things that I know have helped me and others. I am not going to share antibiotic protocols as I am not medically trained to discuss those, and I know some people may have allergic reactions to them. I have taken them on and off throughout my journey.

1. The Cowden Protocol, it's the herbs listed below. You can purchase them here. https://www.nutramedix.com/shop/cowden-support-program/cowden-support-program-month-1

2. The Buhner protocol, you can find information about this protocol here. http://buhnerhealinglyme.com/

3. The salt C protocol

http://thelymespot.blogspot.com/2010/03/adis-saltc-protocol.html

4. The gum spirit protocol

https://archive.org/stream/turp_candida_daniels/turp_candida_daniels_djvu.txt

5. Desbio - They have different vials for different co-infections as well.

6. Essential oils for Lyme-Now here is just a list, you would have to investigate each one and see what you think would work for you. I would not personally ingest these or any essential oil without a carrier oil like coconut oil or olive oil myself.

oregano oil thieves

cinnamon bark, Spearmint

clove bud tea tree

garlic marjoram

cinnamon bark peppermint

allspice breath

myrrh palmarosa

hydacheim eucalyptus

Litsea cubeba amyris

Geranium cumin

patchouli dark comment

lavender cedarwood

clary sage

There is also a protocol called a Lyme bullet which uses three oils usually with a carrier oil, I have tried some of these in the past. Since I react to everything it was too much for me but it may help others. Lyme bullet uses thieves' oil, oregano oil, and frankincense oil.

For myself, I have had Lyme for a long time. At least 8 years now to get the Lyme out of my brain. We used IV antibiotics for 28 days. I believe this in addition to the herbals I have taken on and off for the last almost 8 years is what has helped me the most. I am going to also list the things I take at the end of this chapter for people to research to see if they can help them as well.

Now some of the things I am going to list you may think I am not going to do this or try that, and that is okay. These are things I had to use and still use to get myself well. We must be our advocate with Lyme, no one is coming to save us, we must save ourselves and then share how we did it to save everyone else. At least that has always been my thoughts on this.

Constipation- I use mag 07, I use enemas, the regular one, and coffee ones. This also helps get rid of dead toxins killed off from medicine.

Pain- I use LDN, and Cannabis (I have a medical MJ card, and tend to use RSO oil or feco)

If you don't have access to this, I would try a good CBD oil as it helps anxiety and pain

Mast Cell Amazing Nutrition- Quercetin 800 Mg with Bromelain 165

Mg- Amazon

Metalation issues- L methionine from Now products, and Heapto synergy from apex energetics

(The Heapto opens 3 pathways and allows the toxins to come out in your urine)

Thyroid- I use GTA -Forte 11 by biotics research

Fish oil- for inflammation I use any non-GMO kind up to 6 grams a day

Adrenals-Apex Energetics – AdrenaCalm (KR-16) 1.6Oz

Parasite – Mimosa Pudica organic-Amazon

Detox the brain- Neuro-Antitox II CNS/PNS-https://www.jnutra.com/ (it's cheapest here)

Binding- Activated charcoal, GI detox, there are quite a few of these, look into them and see what you think may help you.

Detox the liver- Milk thistle, liver support by vital nutrients

Detox the Lymph Nodes-Red Root cleanse and detoxify by herb & pharm-Amazon

Detox the skin-Epsom salt baths

For the heart- I get chest pain so I use Acetyl L -carnitine

Vitamins- Vitamin D with food, potassium pill by Now products, for some reason I can't seem to handle any B vitamins even if they are methylated b vitamins

For my mental health- Music, movies, and prayer

Now here is a treatment plan that I am going to suggest, and each thing should be looked at and considered. We all have different co-infections so some of these things that work for me may not work for you.

I am going to suggest them anyway. I am in no way a doctor; I am just suggesting you to look into to see if this could help you too.

Mthfr Genes-I have two Mthfr Genes which means for me I can't detox on my own. This is a big reason I was having over 20 seizures a day when I first became sick. We were trying to kill the Lyme, but the toxins had nowhere to go, so they just dumped it back in my bloodstream. This is an issue for so many people with Lyme and they just don't know it. I would check to see if your detox pathways are working before trying anything. I mean anything for Lyme treatment. If you don't you will most likely herx like crazy. I received my test from Labcorp, it's called the MTHFR test. So, for me, if I meet someone newly bit my advice is to make sure you can detox properly, and that your pathways are open. If they are not there are things you can do to help your body get rid of toxins. If you're not detoxing, I would look into a product I suggested before called heapto synergy as it helps open three pathways.

Kill Lyme- It's your choice what you use to kill it. There are different things you can try like herbals, antibiotics, and there is even new medicine like Dapsone and Disulfiram. I have tried many different things to kill Lyme and I felt for my brain the IV antibiotics and then the herbals I have listed went with it is what helped the most. I know people that have gotten well with just herbals. I personally think that antibiotics and herbals are what works the best for me, but I haven't been able to try any of the new medicines like Dapsone, and Disulfiram. There are also essential oils that have been shown to kill Lyme in various stages, and I listed those in a different chapter. Some people also use rife, but I am not familiar with this as I have never been able to afford one.

Binders-Once your detox pathways are open you are ready to start treating. It's your choice how you want to treat it. I believe that everyone should be binding. So, what I mean is you take the medicine to kill the Lyme then you wait about two to three hours before you bind, some doctors will suggest you sweat first then you bind. This is okay if you're healthy enough to make yourself sweat. When I first became sick I could not sweat at all, and doing anything physical such as walking was too much for me. So, if you can't sweat on your own I would do a detox bath with Epsom salt, then take the binder. This is just my suggestion, and I have found it to help me.

Binders part 2-Now when it comes to binding there are many choices from activated charcoal to Gi Detox, a product that some of the doctors talk about. My go-to is always activated charcoal and sometimes I even use GI detox. You can go online and type in binders and see which one you think may work for you. Now there are prescription binders like Csm or Cholestyramine. I have used this binder and for me, it was too strong. There is also one called Welcol that is also a prescription if you're doing this on your own. Getting these medicines may be impossible so I am going to tell you how to bind without these. I would use something like bentonite clay, activated charcoal, chlorella, zeolite or pectin. I use activated charcoal and chlorella, and if I am binding mold I use Gi Detox. Just make sure when binding, to take it away from any other medicines. So, I will take something to kill like antibiotics, wait two hours then I take a detox bath, and after the bath, I normally will take some activated charcoal. This way it binds whatever I am killing off and it helps reduce the chance for a herx reaction.

Parasites-As you're killing off Lyme and these other co-infections you will also have to kill parasites. People say "well, I don't have parasites," but if you have Lyme you have parasites. If you read my first book you will see all the things I have killed since getting Lyme. I use mimosa pudica for this. I have also used other things like goat dewormer, MMS, and other herbal parasite medicines. I find Mimosa pudica to be the best if you can't get a hold of a prescription parasite medicine, which for me I have never been able to afford one, or get them from a doctor. Be very careful of MMS, as it gave me a stomach infection and landed me in the ER. No one explained how dangerous this could be. I know this doesn't happen to everyone, but I would use caution when considering buying and using this.

When killing parasites you need to think of it as cleaning up your house, your house is your body. I do monthly maintenance around the full moon cycle and I normally will start it three days before the moon and keep going three days after the new moon or full moon. I was doing this every day, but now that I have them under control I do monthly maintenance to make sure they don't come back.

So, we talked about killing Lyme, binding toxins, and killing parasites. Now we need to look at our whole bodies and see how the Lyme is affecting it. Depending on what is going on with your symptoms is how I would treat the disease.

I think most people with Lyme should be on fish oil if they can take it, it lowers inflammation and when inflammation goes down so does our pain.

Teeth-I had a lot of issues with my teeth. I had mercury fillings and that was causing me to not heal. So, if you are like me you're going to have to get this taken care of, it's just one more part of the puzzle. I recommend seeing a biomedical dentist so the mercury doesn't go back into your bloodstream or mouth.

Brain and Brain Fog- If you're like me and you suffer from brain fog you will need to detox your brain as well. I use a product that I listed before called neuro antitox 11 CNS pns, it detoxes the brain. I would start slow and build up. I also suggest taking a binder a few hours after taking this to make sure you soak up any toxins. I also use high dose fish oil for this. Find you a nice, cheap non-gmo fish oil and start out low, and go up. I take about 6mgs a day, and it has lowered my inflammation.

Herx- Sometimes no matter what you take you herx. If you're in a herx, or having a herx reaction; that could be pain, burning, throwing up, and/or a slight fever. People will experience different things with a herx. I have a few products that I consider my go-to. I use bur bur pinella by nutramedix. If I am herxing really bad I will step up the binding and detoxing. There have been times where I have had to take up to five baths a day. I do recommend anyone with Lyme that doesn't have heat intolerance to think about getting a heating blanket. I am on my third one I think in the last 7 or 8 years. I swear it has helped me, the heat seems to help when the pain is so bad I want to go crazy.

Also Alka seltzer gold will help with a herx reaction, I buy it from Cvs online.

Mental state- Let's face it, if you have Lyme you have experienced some depression, anxiety, maybe even some depersonalizing. It's almost like we don't even recognize ourselves or our bodies anymore. I remember when I was super sick I had no memory of my childhood. It was almost like I didn't know the memories were there. My childhood was rough. I won't go into details about it here, but it probably is one reason I have so much trauma in my life. For me when I get depressed or angry or sad, I turn to what I love. Music. Now for you, it may be something else like knitting or drawing, or even watching tv. If you're in a bad mental state I suggest reaching out to someone else with Lyme and have them talk you through it if you feel comfortable with that.

Tremors and Neurological symptoms – I use magnesium for the tremors, and I have tried different kinds.

I tend to use **Magnesium glycinate** as it seems to absorb better. I also use CBD oil for this. I use one called Harlequin CBD and it's high CBD, very low THC, and it seems to help most of the time. There is no magic bullet to any of this stuff, it's mostly trial and error.

Heavy metals- I have had heavy metal numbers come out high since I have had Lyme. I found that zeolite or a spray called TRS to help with this. I bought it online from a local person here that has Lyme and I have found it to help. It's your choice how you want to deal with the heavy metals, but in my opinion this is something you will also have to deal with to help fix the body. Just one more piece of the puzzle.

Mold- I use biocidin for this as a kill for mold toxins, then I am using GI detox to mop up the toxins. It's more of a kill, sweat, bind. So for me, I kill with biocidin, bind with GI Detox and sweat with a sauna or bath. It's also important to make sure that your liver is functioning right, and your liver numbers should be checked throughout any of these treatments. Especially for mold and Lyme.

Liver- For the liver, I use milk thistle. I have used liver detox medicine before, and I have even done a liver cleanse. I like the heapto synergy for this as well. It helps detox the liver as well as open pathways.

Chest pain- I have had my heart checked a few times, but they have never found anything wrong with it. Acetyl L -carnitine it the name of the medicine I use, and it's made by different companies. I have used different brands and have had success with it.

Constipation- This is a problem quite a few Lyme patients have. They do not eliminate waste as they should be. We should be going to the bathroom at least two to three times a day. This has been an ongoing issue for me. I like Mag 07 for this, and I have also used a medicine called fiber flow. I also will do enemas, either organic coffee ones or regular ones. There is a group on Facebook called bottoms up and it will teach you how to do the enemas if you're not sure how to do them. Some of the pictures on there are very graphic so if you have a weak stomach this may not be the site for you.

Move your body- Now some Lyme patients are bedridden so they can't get up and walk, I understand that, I was that person. When I was stuck in the bed I would try and make my arms strong so this way I could use them to move my body when my legs didn't work. If you can, move your body every single day. Even if that means just walking a little. I know it hurts, but it's something I feel we must do because if we don't our body forgets how to move and work. When I was in a wheelchair I used arm weights, and I would use weights on my legs trying to get them to become stronger.

Mast cell- Mast cells can do different things to your body; some people become allergic to foods, for me I became allergic to my environment. Anything scented would set me off. If someone was wearing perfume or cologne, if their shampoo was scented, it would cause me to have tremors and my face would flush and burn. One time we washed our clothes in Glade laundry soap as it was bought by mistake. I wasn't the one that washed the clothes, and when I put the shirt on my throat started to close as if someone was choking the life out of me. Over the years I have tried many different mast cell medicines. I even did the h1/h2 antihistamines. It made me very tired and I couldn't get out of bed. So I kept researching and watching summits until I found the mold summit. They talked about how if you have Lyme and Mold, lots of times you have chemical sensitivity and Mast cells. I found this product to work the best for me: Amazing Nutrition-Quercetin 800 Mg with Bromelain 165 Mg- I buy it from Amazon. It's a really good product. I take two first thing when I get up in the morning, I should be taking it three times a day, but money is always tight and if I can spread out my medicine, I try to.

Seizures- Now I have two different kinds of seizures: one kind I am completely aware of what is happening to me, I just can't talk or do anything about them. The other, and I have only had these a few times throughout this Lyme stuff, will have me foaming from my mouth completely out of it, and I hate to admit this but I have even soiled myself once during a really bad one. I think they are called grand mal seizures. I have tried like three or four different seizures meds, but they did not help me at all, I changed my diet, went keto genetic, and still, the seizure remained. The only thing that seems to help stop them is to make sure I take my medicine for the mast cell.

DNR's- For people that don't know what this is, it's Dvd that helps retrain your brain. I am in no way saying this is all in our heads, it's not. The Dvd helps us to not be stimulated by our environments. I have been trying to get it for the last few years. I never really had the extra 300 dollars it cost to buy it. A friend of mine here in Illinois had her own and borrowed it to me. She is an amazing friend that is sick herself. She has even brought me medicine before when I couldn't afford to see another doctor get some.

Tests I have used over the years to watch my number and help me improve.

Now I normally test through quest as my insurance will cover most of them, and it's very important to try and get some of your testing covered. Having Lyme is already so expensive that if we can cut some of the cost that will only help us. Plus, what I don't spend on tests I can spend on medicine.

The testing I think most people would agree on is having your vitamin levels checked, especially vitamin D and B12.

Another test is the test for inflammation levels called the HS CRP, my numbers used to be so high with this, and as I killed off a lot of the Lyme and co-infections my numbers have gone down to normal. I also take high doses of fish oil that helps lower these numbers.

Also, ebv, and co-infection tests, Now some of the testing's are not that great, like Bart tests. Just remember that if you ask to take any of the co-infection tests they are about as good as a Lyme test, in my opinion, about a 50/50 chance you will get accurate results.

Thyroid panel

Another testing to see if you can detox, Mthfr testing

In the past, I have had a C4a test done to check for toxins, but insurance is really picky about covering it, so I stopped asking for that test.

People with Lyme lots of time will have insulin issues. My glucose will go high, then drop low, so getting your ALT and glucose tests are done, in my opinion, is worth the money. If you don't want to take prescription medicine, that has a lot of side effects, there are herbal medicines that can help lower these numbers and keep them more on the normal side.

Chapter 09

Burning Mouth Syndrome

In the middle of January, my mouth started to burn. At first, I thought it was a tooth, but then the gums and all the teeth started to hurt too. It feels like my mouth is on fire, the same fire that I have had in the past in my legs, and head. Somehow what's left of the Lyme is attacking my mouth. I can feel it, I know what's happening, I have been here too many times not to understand it. I would be lying if I said this disease didn't drive me crazy. It's horrible how much pain it causes. People say oh yes, this person has a little case of Lyme. Huh? There is no little case of this crap, you either have it or you don't and if you have it, it's horrible.

Do you know what happened in the '90s with the Hiv/Aids patients? They were so sick, and no one wanted to help them so they had to help themselves. I feel like that is how we are treated with Lyme. They don't understand our disease, so they tend to ignore us. We are left on our own, trying to figure out how to get ourselves out of pain and fewer symptoms when it's hard for us to think straight, from one minute to the next.

On January 29th I went to the dentist here in Villa Park, and the dentist diagnosed me with burning mouth syndrome. She said it was from Lyme Disease. She gave me some medicine to numb my mouth, but it didn't work. So here I go again researching how to help myself. I gave up coffee, yes me the person that can drink five cups a day. I literally couldn't drink it, it made my mouth burn worse. I learned that cayenne pepper helps stop the mouth from burning, so I bought a liquid organic kind from amazon and along with some cayenne pills, mixed with some CBD oil, and I have found that it is helping.

A week later my tooth started to hurt, and I went to get it pulled out only to find out it's infected. So now I am on another week of antibiotics to clear the infection. If it's not one thing it's another. It's cold and snowy here in Illinois today. I am so ready for Spring, I can't complain though this winter hasn't been too bad. Heck we stayed above 30 degrees most of the time.

I found out online that we can buy medicine from overseas that we can't get a hold of here in Illinois. I probably could get some here if I had money to pay for a doctor, but I am out of money, so I am doing what I need to do. The medicine is called Disulfiram. We have to be careful about this medicine. Someone, a doctor or an fnp, needs to follow your progress on this and check your numbers, liver, etc. I know all of this as I have been researching it. I do have more good days than bad days now, but I am still not 100 percent. I am not telling you to go buy medicine overseas. What I am saying is I have had enough with Lyme and I am desperate enough to try it. So, for me, this is what I am going to do. We have been going back and forth with this decision for months, finally, I chose to order some online.

There are a lot of precautions that must be taken when using this type of medicine; you can't have any alcohol in your system at all, even skincare products or hair products. So, this is something I have to make sure I remember as some of our products that I have used in the past for Lyme have an alcohol base.

Chapter 10

Disulfiram

Disulfiram- It's a medicine to treat alcoholism but has been shown in some studies to kill persistent forms of Lyme Disease.

So, I have been researching this medicine for the last year. I am very interested in trying it, but I couldn't get a doctor to let me. So I did what I had to do and I found a way to order it online. Yep, we have reached the point where I have to do what I need to to recover completely. I have been at this for almost 8 years, if someone would have told me back in 2012/2013 or even 2014 that I would still be here, I would say, I hope so. I never thought I would make it this far in my life with Lyme. I was super sick, I remember being bedridden, being wheelchair-bound, and needing a walker. I remember when I couldn't put on my socks when I needed help to make it to the washroom. I have come extremely far, but I am not where I want to be, I want to be working full time.

My brain did clear up a lot after the Iv antibiotics so I will be forever grateful for Dr. T because he did that for me. I just know this part; the rest of my healing is going to be up to me. I am forever researching, and I was looking for ways to improve my immune system. With these viruses and things going around, we all need to be a little more cautious. So, I have been trying to laugh more, it's good for the immune system and get enough sleep. I know these things are very important.

So, this is going to be my protocol. I may tweak it here and there. I am going to start with 1/8 of a pill, my pills are 250 mg. I am going to take it with some taurine, and some Dihydromyricetin, and L- ornithine. The taurine is for the nerves, the L-ornithine is to get the ammonia out, and then the Dhm is in case I accidentally ingest anything with alcohol in it. I will also be taking things to detox like heapto synergy, Epsom salt baths, and GI detox for a binder. I am going to start slow and see how I do. I will also add in the tick recovery, it's a herbal you can find on amazon. I am doing that because I have bart and it will come out once we start going after the Lyme. This is going to be my protocol and along with that, I will get my liver checked about every four weeks or so. This is not going to be a long-term treatment. I am going to start every three days, and do that for about two months and see how I do. If I see improvement but still have lingering symptoms I will continue with the treatment a little longer. I am the experiment, I am the person that needs to get well, so I must be prepared to do this.

There are a lot of precautions that must be taken when using this type of medicine; you can't have any alcohol in your system at all, even skin care products or hair products. So, this is something I have to make sure I remember as some of our products that I have used in the past for Lyme have an alcohol base.

Day 1

March 4th, 2020

Disulfiram

Now I am the type of person to research well before I try something. I wasn't that way in the past and my body paid dearly for that. So before I started this, a few days ago I started to open up my detox pathway with heapto synergy (APEX ENERGETICS)

On Wednesday when I decided to start the meds I had previously taken Diflucan for yeast just in case. I had already brought alcohol-free products from shampoo to body soap and hand soap. I looked through my herbals to make sure which ones were safe and which weren't on this protocol. I also went on Disulfiram.net, to learn the ins and outs of this medicine. By safe I mean alcohol-free. When I started, I thought I could go up to 250 quickly. I didn't realize how strong this medicine is. So, I started on 1/8 of a 250 mg pill, so 31.25. I had already purchased some l-ornithine to get the ammonia out of the body, some zinc, and some Molybdenum. I am also on LDN nightly, so I had to investigate how medicine interacts with each other. I recommend everyone doing this; check your medicines just in case. Then I called my FNP so that I could get a liver check-up, and have my blood tests done. It recommends doing it before and about 7 -14 days afterward just in case, as sometimes this medicine will raise the liver enzymes. It's something we have to watch carefully.

Day 2

March 5th, 2020

No killing medicine today, I just focused on detox. Last night I felt burning in places I never burned before, like my elbows. So I know this is working, but I have to go slow. I did a sauna, just a cheap pop up one I had my daughter buy for me. I was in it for 20 minutes, then I took a cold shower for 3 minutes to wipe off the toxins. Yes, it sucked, but I was told by a medical clinic here in Lombard that this is the best way to get the toxins off. I drank water all day long, took 3 pills of L-orthine, and then waited before taking some Molybdenum. I also bought some liver support with vital nutrients.

Day 3

March 6th, 2020

I woke up feeling good. I had spurts of energy that I haven't had in a very long time. I knew that I was going to crash. I always do, but I did as much as I could while it lasted. Today I stepped up the detox, I did heapto synergy again, took an Epsom salt bath, and tried to do a self-massage on my lymph nodes because they are hurting. I placed a call to have a lymph massage on Tuesday next week. I need help learning how to do this myself and they will do it, then teach me how to do things at home. I did not take any more of the DSF or Disulfiram because I want to go slow. I disagree with going fast because this stuff is really strong. I think we are all at different levels of our healing and too fast can hurt us. That's just my opinion, I am not a medically trained person. This is just from my own experience. Also, it's going to be a full moon on Monday, so I had to do my monthly parasite kill. I usually start it a day or two before the full moon and go on a day or two after. I have tried different medicines for this but feel that mimosa pudica, the organic kind, works best for me.

Day 4

March 7th, 2020

I woke up with my left index finger being kind of numb. I recognized this as being a sign that I may be experiencing a little neuropathy, so I took some zinc.

Throughout the morning, I was able to go out and do some errands, but my body just felt so achy. I also was very low on energy. I decided to only take the medicine once a week. It's strong, and it kills stuff. Today I did an enema, just a Walgreens kind one, and I saw some biofilm. If you're squeamish, you may want to skip over this part. The stuff that came out is like an orange kind of almost rubble like substance. I think it's very important to make sure you eliminate waste at least two to three times a day, which is difficult because so many of us deal with constipation from Lyme. If you are constipated, try some magnesium or some mag 07, also milk thistle. My head was kind of burning or zapping some. I attribute this to die off. I just rested as much as I possibly could, then I started to feel better. I order some Dihydromyricetin or (DHM) off amazon. This is just in case I inject alcohol by mistake, It shouldn't happen, but sometimes even vinegar will cause a reaction and I would rather be safe than sorry. At least this is what I found while researching.

Day 5

March 8th, 2020

Today I woke up feeling pretty good. Since 2012, mornings have been hard for me. My body doesn't do well in the morning, I normally start to feel better around 1 pm or so. I got up, cleaned, did some homework, and researched some more. One of my big issues is Bart, and I know with this medicine, Bart can come out worse as biofilm is killed off. So right now I am looking to find what to take that will kill Bart. I have seen where some people have used tick recovery which I have here so I think I may just try that unless I can get my hands on some Rifamycin. We will see, most likely it will be something herbal I need to take. The tick recovery I bought off amazon so that may come in handy.

Day6

March 9th, 2020

I overslept today; I didn't wake up until 9 am. It could be because of the time change, we are now into March, or because I was up later than normal last night. Anyway today, I feel a little burning, but nothing too bad. The numbness in my finger is pretty much gone. I added back my fish oil, my metabolic extra, and my glycine today. I take about 3 to 6 grams of fish oil a day to help with inflammation. The other two medicines are to keep my glucose levels down. The burning of my urine has gone away. I believe it's a lot of toxins since I don't have any other pain or fever or anything of that sort. Therefore, I need to go very slow.

Day 7

March 10th, 2020

Today I woke up feeling a little achy, the weather here has been up and down. I had my Lymph massage at 10 am today. I went in a little nervous, but the place in Downers Grove was amazing. She knew so much about Lyme and she did a great number on me. Afterward, my stomach hurt pretty bad then when I urinated the smell that came out of me, was completely toxic. I will find a cheaper place to go, as we can't afford 400 a month for this, not with all the other medicine that I need.

Day 8

03/11/2020

Last night and this morning, I had quite a bit of pain in my stomach then I expelled quite a bit of worm looking parasites. My urine smells like ammonia, so I know that the Lymph massage worked, it's getting the toxins out. I wonder if these parasites hide in the Lymph nodes. After doing some research I found that certain parasites do cause issues with the Lymph nodes, especially ones that come from cats. I have had cats my whole life and took many off the street as kittens, a matter of fact one of the cats I have now we saved as a baby 10 years ago. I always took them to the vet right away, but you never know if I could have picked up something from them as well.

Then I took two weeks off, and will start again, 1/8 of a pill, and just focus on detox. I know this sounds like it wouldn't be effective, but I have been able to do more now than ever before, so it's working, but I am going very slow. Yes, I want the disease out of me, but if I am not well enough to get out of bed then what sense does it make to do it that way. I am learning slowly and steady for me is the way to go. So this is going to be my protocol, only once a month to take the medicine and just detox the rest. I have been sick for a very long time, so I am going to do it this way. So far it's working, and I don't want to mess that up.

April 11th, 2020

Day 1

I had my blood test results yesterday and my liver is a little elevated but nowhere as bad as it has been in the past. So I am going to take 1/8 of a tablet again. I wanted to make sure my liver was okay to proceed, I know I am taking a lot of precautions, but I feel like I must. I am also making sure I have no alcohol in my system at all. I don't drink but I mean in any product. I also need to stay away from vinegar as for some reason with this medicine I react to that too.

I will start again soon, just going to focus again on detoxing, slow and steady for me is the way to go. I seem to get better when I do things this way, compared to when I take too much medicine at once and try to kill too much off at once.

Chapter 11

Here and Now

We are now in January of 2020. Yes baby, I made it another year. I am going to be 44 years old this year. Some people hate to get older, but for me, I welcome it, I love it. It means one more year to spend with the people I love, one more sunset, one more day to love my kids, husband and family. I am starting to have a lot more good days than bad, but I still have some symptoms that come and go. For instance, today the nerves in my legs started to jump and they were visible through my jeans. It burns when this happens, this is a symptom that can spoil a nice day.

People ask me this all the time; how do I remain such a positive person? If you read my first book you would know that for a long time with Lyme I was in a dark place.

Some days when my ears would ring and the light would hurt my eyes, I would just lay in my bed and cry. I didn't understand what was happening to me, and I blamed myself for not realizing it sooner. I felt every emotion a person can feel; I felt like a failure, a burden, I couldn't even keep my house clean. One day it just hit me that the world wouldn't expect someone that was as sick with a different disease to do all of this. So why am I so hard on myself?

My life has become quite busy with the family moving closer and I am more involved than ever before. Even with school and everything going on in my life I still yearn to work. It's like part of myself is missing, has been missing for almost 8 years because of Lyme. I miss getting up, dressing up and going to work. I miss having a paycheck and responsibility. I miss it all. I keep telling myself I am getting close, I just have to get a few more symptoms under control. The disabled people told me that to be able to work a person has to go a whole month without missing any work due to illness. At this point a few days a month I am still down, I mean those days my symptoms are too bad and I can't do what I need to. Usually, these symptoms are seizures or pain, but I am getting them more and more under control.

I still research when I can, taking notes. I am trying to help myself get into remission and stay that way. We are now into May 2020 and I started thinking that I am now able to try and find something, a part-time job. I still have mast cell, Lyme and co-infections but the medicine I am on is allowing me to have fewer seizures from perfumes and other scents. So, I started to look for something part-time at home, a legit job that I could do to make some extra money. Let's face it, having Lyme is very expensive. The herbal medicines alone will cost a fortune, not to mention all the credit I have used the past few years trying to survive this disease. I have to pay it all back, and disability just does not cover much at all. I started to look at online job places like Upwork, and I put in a few jobs to work at home. Last night I received a message that someone is interested in me to do some collections at home for them. It would only be very part-time but for me, this is a big step. I haven't worked since January of 2013. I didn't get that job, but it was good practice interviewing again.

If you have stumbled on to my story online or if you have Lyme yourself or are reading this so you can help someone you love, please remember to be patient. This disease is not a one pill fix, all our bodies are different and what my body can handle yours may not be able to. So, my advice is no matter what you're going to try to go slow. I also believe in only starting one new thing at one time because if you're going to react and you're on different medicines it will be too hard to decide which one is the one that is causing the issue. Again, anything I say in the book should not be taken as medical advice, I am in no way a doctor. I am just giving you my advice from my own experiences with Lyme, Mold, Mast Cell, and Co-infections.

Today is a warmer Illinois day, with a hint of spring in the air. It's supposed to get 65 today. I love warmer weather. I tend to do better in spring, and summer then I do in the wintertime. If it falls below 30 degrees or so my bones ache. It wasn't this way before Lyme, it's just how it is now after Lyme. If I can give anyone new to Lyme or even anyone reading this book some advice, I would say, don't be so hard on yourself. I know you want to be well; I understand it more than most people, but if we push ourselves too fast, or too much, we can and will go backward. I am a perfect example of this. So, for now, I go slow and steady.

With me it's not just Lyme, it's Lyme, and mold, that triggered mast cell, parasites, and co-infections, especially Bart. I realized even though I hit Bart with antibiotics, I still have it, how do I know that? Well, my feet burn like crazy at times. My brain gets these zaps, and my body has inner tremors or vibrations. It's not every day, but it's still there, not as bad as it was, as I did treat Bart already with some antibiotics. We used azithromycin. I think I am going to treat the rest with herbals, as abx or antibiotics messed up my gut and gave me yeast issues the last time I was on them.

I mentioned in the past I am on a freelance site. Well, with all this craziness going on, I started to get little jobs. So, I am hoping to work part-time now. I am hoping to land a job for about 20-30 hours a week at home. For now, I am taking whatever is given to me. With any site you must be careful, I never bid on jobs that don't have any reviews, as I have done that in the past, and they have turned up to be scams. So, for me, I have a process when I am on this site; I look for money that has been paid out, and reviews. I wouldn't go to a doctor or restaurant without checking the reviews so why would I for a job.

So today I was given a job, I found it through Upwork, it's a job entering a number in excel. I can do it at home, and it will help. My husband still works as much as possible, but times right now are hard. Places are cutting hours, things are closing, it's a very scary time. I am just grateful to be working. It's exciting and what I have wanted to do for the last 7, almost 8 years. Amazingly, I was able to do this job when for a very long time I couldn't even get out of bed, I couldn't sit up, my brain wouldn't even allow me to read. I remember a time, when I was researching, I had to lay down after every few minutes, I just couldn't do it. I am so close, but I am not cured, I even wonder if I will ever be fully cured. If I can have a life, I can accept that though.

Chapter 12

The Coronavirus

The last few weeks have been crazy, our schools have closed, all sports events are either on hold or done for the season. They even stop the courts from going into session. This virus started in China and made its way here to the United States, at least that is what the news is saying. I tend to take everything I hear with a grain of salt. Our friends at the CDC, I used that word friend because it's ironic, has told everyone to stock up on two weeks of food, and necessities.

03/20/2020

Today Illinois went on a stay at home order by our governor. We can go to the grocery store, to the bank, to hospitals, doctors, laundromat vets, and restaurants, but we can't socialize with anyone and we should be standing 6 feet away from everyone. We can go in our yard too, so it's not as horrible as it sounds. The worst thing is all the people being without work, I worry they won't be able to survive. Plus, lots of the stores are without inventory, how will babies eat if there is no food or milk.

We are now on 03/24/2020 we have over 1500 cases of the virus here in Illinois and 16 people have died so far. It's a scary time, everything is closed, the Libraries, to parks, the only things that are still open are called essential businesses. So many are without jobs right now since the hotels and a lot of restaurants have closed. I wear a mask now whenever I go out and that is only to the grocery store. People thought I was nuts a month ago when I brought masks for my family. Now I have strangers walking up to me asking where they can buy one.

Today I went to the grocery store with my mask on and had an elderly lady stop me to ask where I got my mask from. I took down her number, she has cancer, and I went home and brought her a mask to wear too. No one with cancer should have to go without a mask, this should not be happening. I can't afford to get everyone a mask, I am on a fixed income myself, but if I can help one person I will. Listen, I don't know what is going to happen with this virus, but I do know I am trying to prepare my family. We are taking vitamin C, and olive leaf, to try and build our immune systems up. My husband is around quite a few people, so it makes me nervous that he will bring the virus home. I have to protect us at all costs. I know I shouldn't be that scared but I am. I have taken every precaution necessary, I even wear gloves at the store, so I don't touch the keypad or anything with my bare hands.

We are taking extra measures at home to keep ourselves safe. I have everyone on vitamin c, olive leaf, and airborne gummies. We all have a mask and gloves. We only go out if it's necessary too. We have lost something like 16 people already in Illinois due to this virus. I read that there are now like 1535 cases, every country has someone that is sick, if not multiple people. We must stay safe. In the City of Chicago now the police have the authority to break up large groups, the law is not any groups over 8 people. I am not sure why anyone would want to risk their health with this, but some people feel they are immune to it, they are not

We have 30k people infected with COVID-19 here now, and so many deaths. I don't know if people just didn't take the news seriously or what. I know I had people laugh at me when I brought masks two months ago, but I was watching, reading and trying to get ahead of what was coming. Now everyone is wearing masks here, heck most towns it's against the law now to go out without one. It's a scary time for everyone, and if you're not following instructions and social distancing you're part of the problem in my opinion. This won't last forever but we need to try and lower the curve, we already have so many people sick with this virus. I am trying to do what I can to not be part of the problem, but part of the solution.

Today is 04/20/20 and we are still on the stay at home order. Most of the family-owned restaurants, the smaller ones, have closed. Things like hair salons, pet grooming places, nail salons, all closed down for now. It's eerie driving down the street, you barely see anyone or any cars. It's like we are in a movie, it's hard to explain. Then when we do go to the store everyone is in masks now, and people always need to stay 6 feet apart. It's a very strange and scary time.

My heart goes out to all the first responders, the families of essential workers that have to go to work during this scary time. If someone would have told me this was the way it was going to be 6 months ago, I wouldn't have believed you. I did feel this was coming before some people and brought a deep freezer to put food in, just in case we would need it, and let me tell you it has come in handy. We wear masks everywhere now, and all the parks are now closed for kids to play in. Even if you see a family walking down my street now, which is rare, they are all masked up. Even the little ones.

Chapter 13

Living with Lyme

We are on April 20, 2020, and the weather is starting to get warmer finally. With every Spring I get nervous for everyone because some do not know the dangers lurking right in their yards. I had someone reach out to me that lives in the same town and she has Lyme too. It seems more and more are getting infected and less are getting cured, at least that is what I am seeing. At this point where I am at, I am not sure there is a cure, especially if it's been left untreated. I think for me, I just have to try and live the best life I can with this disease. I am better than I ever was throughout this whole almost 8 year period, but I am not cured. I no longer have weeks where I can't get out of bed, I try to get up every single day now, even though some days the pain is hard to deal with. I use each day and go by symptoms, so if like today I woke up and my head feels fuzzy, then I would go to my brain detox medicine, my Nero antitox 11.

Now there are certain things I take every single day no matter what, that is the medicine for mast cell, and my L methionine, fish oil, thyroid medicine, and blood sugar herbs. These I can't miss but depending on my symptoms that day depends on what else I may take. If I feel the Lyme is attacking or I am having a flare, I will go to tick recovery herbal meds or maybe even the Disfiram. If I do take the Antabuse or Disfiram, I must make sure I didn't ingest anything with alcohol in it. Also, anything with vinegar, it will make my head hurt.

I have tried to limit as much stress as possible in my life, that is hard with a pandemic going on, but I am trying. I try to take walks when I can, sometimes I can make it all the way, sometimes I can't, but at least I am trying every single day. My husband and I try to laugh more and have fun more. For a long time, he saw me as a sick wife, and I saw him as my caregiver. Any relationship is already hard, but if one partner is sick, especially with something like Lyme, it can be very hard on the relationship and the whole family. It's not just the one with Lyme that suffers, everyone in the family suffers too. For a long time, I was very angry, the Lyme would make my brain burn so bad, that I felt like it was on fire. Any little noise sounded like it was amplified 1000 times over. The light would hurt my eyes so bad I would cry. I was not a fun person to be around, I was not myself. I am learning each month, each day, to not be that person I was. Now that my symptoms have lessened, for me it was a lot of detoxing, that helped the most, I started to feel like more of myself again.

Even though I am feeling better, I still have to know my limits. I am not a healthy person, so I can't like to go for a run or a 3 to 5-mile walk. Even if it's just something as simple as cleaning the apartment, I have to go slow, and I have to rest. If I am overall tired I take a nap, there is nothing wrong with letting our bodies rest. If I know the next day is going to be difficult I try to rest more the day before. If I am feeling stressed out I will watch a funny show or movie, and just try to relax. I still do my Epson salt baths, and I believe they help. We have to know the limits of our bodies, and we have to listen to our bodies.

If you're just going through Lyme or if you have had it a long time, I want to say, you will get better, just hang in there. It may happen overnight, and it may take years like it has for me. The hardest part of this disease I think is that there is no standard treatment or protocol. I found what works for someone else may not work for me, and vice versa. Some things I do think will work for everyone with Lyme is detoxing, however, the way you choose to do that will only help your body. I also believe in supporting your immune system. No matter what you're fighting or going through, if your immune system can't fight back, it will be very difficult to improve.

This month I received my test results and for the first time in years, my inflammation levels are not through the roof, so that tells me what I am doing is working. Please don't be so hard on yourself, I found that I was incredibly hard on myself throughout this whole process. I would compare myself to a healthy person and say why can't I do that? When I think about it, that is ridiculous. Would we expect someone with Cancer to clean their whole house, cook, work, exercise, and everything else that is expected of a person with Lyme? No, we wouldn't, so I don't like this anymore.

I do what I can, and I rest when I need to, I am not just talking about physically, I am talking about mental rests too. If the news upsets you, shut it off, and listen to some music. If a family member stresses you out, maybe take a step back, and put some distance between the two of you. I know this can be hard, but for our wellbeing, we need to put ourselves first. Try to find something to look forward to every single day, this will get you up and moving. The longer we are in bed the harder it is to get our muscles working. At least I found this to be true for me. I had the hardest time after being stuck in bed for nine months to be able to walk without pain.

I also wanted to remind you that you are not alone, there are millions of people with Lyme, and if you feel like you are, or that you can't take it anymore, reach out to someone, reach out to me, I will try to help you. As I did in my last book, I will have my contact information available at the end of this book. This disease is fighting, and ever-changing, what it does to our bodies and our minds is horrible. We need to try and help each other. I have always tried to share what has helped me so that others do not have to go through years of pain like I had to. Stay strong my Lyme Warriors and fight like your life depends on it, because it really does…..

Tera

60

I was born in Chicago and spent time back and forth between Illinois and West Virginia. I never considered myself a city girl, I am country at heart. I am a mother, a wife, a sister, a daughter, and a pet lover. I am currently enrolled at NLU getting my BA degree in Human Services. My goal is to get my degree and help disabled people like myself who had an event or disease disable them.

Contact me

As I stated before and, in this book, you can reach me by a few ways. I am on Facebook, twitter, and Instagram.

F/B -https://www.facebook.com/tera.banks.7

Twitter-https://twitter.com/4mylymewarrior

Instagram-https://www.instagram.com/ts.bankslyme/

You can also email me directly at terabanks4508@gmail.com